Home Remedies

For Constipation

And Diarrhea

Home Remedies
For Constipation
And Diarrhea

By Monica Sidoine,
S.N.H.S. Dip. Herbalism

DISCLAIMER

This book is to serve as an informational guide for use in the home. The remedies and procedures contained in this book are meant to supplement and are not intended to be a substitute for professional medical care. Please seek a qualified medical practitioner for all ailments. The author nor distributors takes no responsibility for customers choosing to treat themselves. Your use of this information is at your own risk.

ISBN - 13: 978-1533562609
ISBN - 10: 1533562601

Proof Read by Jasmine Ned Anunda

Printed By Create Space Publishing
United States of America

ACKNOWLEDGMENTS

I would like to thank all those who have contributed in one way or another to the completion of HOME REMEDIES FOR CONSTIPATION AND DIARRHEA.

I thank God for giving me the vision, wisdom and good health to write this book. For all he has done and will continue to do in my life.

For the many prayer warriors who interceded on behalf of this project and also their moral support.

I thank my daughter Jasmine Ned Anunda for proof reading.

Thank you all.

Monica Sidoine.

PREFACE

The procedures in this Book was designed to be as simple as possible so that anyone will be able to follow them. Most of the items used are local things which you would either have at home, in your kitchen garden or can be easily purchased from the local market or health store for a very low cost.

TABLE OF CONTENTS

CONSTIPATION

Constipation is a condition in which a person or animal has difficulty in eliminating solid waste from the body and the feces are hard and dry.

There are two different types of constipation:-
Organic - this form of constipation requires your doctor's immediate attention.
Functional - with this form of constipation we are in control.

Organic constipation happens when the body undergoes some sort of physical change, like an obstruction or deformation in the colon.

Functional constipation occurs when we are not eating a well-balanced diet, not drinking the right fluids in appropriate quantities, living a high stress life, living an improper lifestyle for our body's well-being.

Some factors which can lead to constipation are:-

- Consuming, and therefore absorbing, an excessive amount of toxins in the body.
- Depression and stress.
- Remaining bedridden.
- Suffering from colitis, or a spastic colon.
- A side effect of diabetes.
- Diverticulosis or tumors of the rectum or anus.
- Drinking caffeinated beverages like coffee, tea, and sodas.
- For certain people consuming milk.
- Eating too much protein.
- Ingesting refined sugars.

- Consuming too much food in one sitting.
- Excessive contact with organophosphate insecticides.
- Excessive usage of iron supplements.
- Over use of enemas.
- Excessive use of certain seasonings.
- Excess amounts of calcium in the body.
- Lethargy.
- Sensitivity to specific foods
- Elevated body temperature – A high fever can cause the colon to accumulate warmth and harden stools.
- A side effect from hypothyroidism -
  Reduced levels of your thyroid hormones.
- Irritable Bowel Syndrome.
- Kidney failure.
- Not enough good bacteria in your gut.
- Insufficient amounts of essential minerals.
- Nerve damage in your digestive tract.
- Not thoroughly chewing food.
- Inadequate fluid intake.
- Leading a sedentary lifestyle and not exercising.
- Premenstrual tension.
- Advanced age.
- Overeating.
- Abuse of laxatives.
- Taking too much Vitamin D.
- Parasites.
- Inadequate digestion.
- Delaying a bowel movement.
- Pregnancy.
- Spinal injury – Certain injuries can harm the nerves that control bowel moments.
- Hepatotoxicity – Toxic liver.
- Use of certain prescription drugs.
- Other various diseases.

NATURAL REMEDIES

- Drink two cups of slightly hot water with 1 lime juice and half a teaspoon of salt added to it.

- Add 1 teaspoon of sea salt to 1 ½ cups of water. Bring it to a boil, allow it to get warm.
  Drink it in the morning.

- Combine 1 tablespoon of flaxseed oil with 1 glass of orange juice along with the pulp and drink it.

- Combine the juice of 1 lemon with 1 cup of warm water and drink it.

- Steep ½ teaspoon of senna leaves to 1 cup of boiling water for 15 minutes.
  Take 1 cup twice daily.

- Steep 1oz of cinnamon in 1 liter of boiling water for 20 minutes.
  Drink 1 cup twice daily for as long as you feel it is necessary.

- Steep 1oz of chamomile in 1 liter of boiling water for 20 minutes.
  Drink 1 cup twice daily for as long as you feel it is necessary.

- Boil 1oz of watermelon seeds in 1 liter of water for 10 minutes. Drink 1 cup twice daily.

- Drink 1 glass of apple juice with lemon or carrot juice first thing in the morning daily.

- Stir 1 teaspoon baking soda in ¼ cup of warm water and drink it.

- Deseed and chop 2 apples and 2 avocados. Blend along with 1 cup of coconut milk and 2 tablespoons of honey until very smooth. Serve cold.

- Mix 2 tablespoons of molasses in 1 cup of warm water and drink it just before bedtime.

- Combine 1 tablespoon of molasses and 1 tablespoon of honey. Take it daily.

- Stir 1 tablespoon of psyllium husk in a glass of water with some lemon juice added to it. Allow it to rest for 5 minutes. Drink it at bedtime.

- Combine 1/8 teaspoon cayenne pepper and 2 cloves of minced garlic with 2 tablespoons of molasses.

- Drink 2oz of aloe juice twice daily.

- Drink 1 cup of aloe juice when the need arises.

- Combine 1 glass of fruit juice with 2 tablespoons of aloe gel. Drink it first thing in the morning.

- Combine 1 glass of grapefruit juice with 2 tablespoons aloe gel.
  Drink it first thing in the morning.
  Then drink 1 teaspoon of coconut oil immediately.

- Steep ½oz of fennel in ½ liter of boiling water for 30 minutes.
  Take 1 cup twice a day.

- Combine ½ teaspoon of ground roasted fennel seeds in 1 cup of warm water.
  Take it daily.

- Steep 3 teaspoons of dried dandelion root in 3 cups of boiling water for 20 minutes.
  Drink 1 cup three times daily.

- Steep 3 teaspoons of dried dandelion leaves in 3 cups of boiling water for 10 minutes.
  Drink 1 cup three times daily.

- Drink 1 tablespoon of olive oil followed by a glass of warm water first thing in the morning.

- Mix 1 teaspoon lemon juice and 1 tablespoon olive oil together.
  Drink it first thing in the morning on an empty stomach.

- Take 2 tablespoons of castor oil for adults and 2 teaspoons for children first thing in the morning.

- Stir 2 teaspoons of Epsom salts in 1 cup of warm water or fruit juice and drink it. If it's for a child use ½ teaspoon of Epsom salts.
  The dosage can be repeated after 4 hours if there has not been any bowel movement.

- Mix one tablespoon each of honey and lemon juice in a glass of warm water.
  Drink it every morning on an empty stomach.

- Drink a glass of water every 30 minutes.

- Blend 3 stewed prunes and 1 tablespoon flaxseeds in some water.
  Have it every morning with the breakfast.

- Soak 12 prunes in 1 cup of water overnight.
  Consume them along with the water that has remained.
  Do this for 8 days.

- Soak 3 almonds and 3 dried figs in some water for a few hours. Grind them into a paste.
  Consume it with 1 tablespoon of honey at nights.

- Drink a glass of prune juice three times daily.

- Drink a glass of coconut milk three times daily.

- Take 1 tablespoon of ground flaxseeds three times daily.

- Mix one tablespoon of flaxseed in a glass of water and allow it to rest for three hours.
  Drink the water daily before bedtime.

- Combine 3 tablespoons of chia seeds, 1 cup coconut milk and 1 teaspoon vanilla essence. Refrigerate overnight.
  Stir and consume.

- Consume ½oz of sesame seeds daily.

- Consume two teaspoons of honey three times a day.

- Increase the intake of fiber in the diet.

- Eat 1 big slice of ripe papaya every morning for breakfast.

- Eat watermelon every morning.

- Eat apples 1 hour after your meals.

- Eat 2 bananas 1 hour after your meals.

- Eat 4oz of raisins daily.

- Have soup as your main meal.

- Eat plenty of green and leafy vegetables and fresh fruits.

- Eat pumpkin, okra, 2 cups of boiled potato leaves, and 7oz of carrots as part of the meal.

- Eat 4 tablespoons of bran daily in the meal.

- Insert 3oz of olive oil in the rectum at nights or rub it on the rectum area.

- Aloe Suppositories - Blend the aloes, put the gel in the fingers of a glove and freeze it.
  Cut into 1" pieces when ready to use and insert it into the rectum.

- Steep 1oz of chamomile in 1 liter of boiling water for 30 minutes. Add it to the water for a cold sitz bath twice a week. See the Hydrotherapy Section.

- Coconut Oil pack.
  See the Hydrotherapy Section.

Health Tips

- Have a balanced diet.

- Avoid eating white flour products.

- Avoid dairy products.

- Avoid meat.

- Get enough sleep and rest daily.

- Do breathing exercises.

- Exercise for at least 30 minutes daily.

- Try to reduce or eliminate the stressors around your lifestyle.

- When the call comes for a bowel movement, do not postpone it for a later time.

DIARRHEA

Diarrhea is frequent and excessive discharging of the bowels producing thin watery feces, usually as a symptom of gastrointestinal upset or infection.

Diarrhea can be acute - lasting one or two weeks, or chronic - continuing for longer than two or three weeks.

Some causes are:-
Bacterial infection.
Food allergies.
Contaminated water.
Food poisoning.
Poor digestion.
Overeating.
Excessive drinking.
Eating too much unripe or overripe fruit.
Eating too much greasy food.
Stress and anxiety.
Side effects of some medications.

Symptoms are:-
Frequent and watery feces.
Abdominal and stomach pains.
Vomiting, thirst, fever, nausea,
Loss of appetite and dehydration.

NATURAL REMEDIES

- Boil 10 young leaves of lemon grass in 2 glasses of water for 10 minutes. Add 1 tablespoon of sugar and 1 small piece of crushed ginger.
  Adults take 1 cup, children 2-6 years ¼ cup, babies 1 tablespoon, 3 times daily and after every loose bowel movement.

- Boil 1oz of ginger in 1 liter of water for 15 minutes.
  Drink 1 cup three times a day.

- Boil 10 chopped guava leaves in 2 glasses of water for 15 minutes.
  Adults take 1 cup, children 2-6 years ¼ cup, 7-12 years ½ cup, babies 1 tablespoon, 3 times daily and after every loose bowel movement.

- Steep 3 teaspoons of chamomile flowers and 3 teaspoons of peppermint leaves in 1 liter of boiling water for 15 minutes.
  Drink 1 cup three times a day.

- Mix one teaspoon each of dried ginger powder, cumin powder, cinnamon powder, and honey.
  Take it three times a day.

- Combine one teaspoon of fenugreek seeds and one tablespoon of roasted cumin seeds in two tablespoons of yogurt.
  Eat it three times a day.

- Combine 1 teaspoon of fenugreek seeds with 1 tablespoon of yogurt.
  Eat it three times a day.

- Have two bananas daily with your breakfast.

- **Severe diarrhea in an adult:** –
  Add 2 large heaping spoonful's of powdered charcoal to a glass of water.
  Drink 1 glass of charcoal water plus 1 glass of plain water 4 times daily. Drink 1 more glass of charcoal water followed by 1 glass of water for each additional watery stool. Use ½ of the dose for a child.

- Steep 1oz of peppermint in 1 liter of boiling water for 30 minutes. Take 1 cup 3 times daily.

- Steep 1oz of red rose petals in 1 liter of boiling water for 30 minutes.
  Take 5 cups daily sweetened with honey.

- Steep 1oz of pomegranate leaves in 1 liter of boiling water for 30 minutes.
  Take 1 spoonful every hour till it stops.

- Steep ½ cup of almond leaves and bark in 1 liter of boiling water for 30 minutes.
  Drink 1 cup twice daily.

- Steep 2 slices of lemon rounds in 2 cups of boiling water for 20 minutes. Strain and add 2 teaspoons of sugar.
  Drink 1 hot cup 3 times daily.

- Take 2 cups of cashew fruit juice daily.

- Take 1 cup of carrot juice daily.

- Drink lots of water.

- Mix 3 tablespoons carob powder in enough water to make a thin paste or put in your oatmeal at breakfast.
  Take ¼ cup 3 times a day at meals.

- Mash 1 ripe banana and add 1 teaspoon of tamarind pulp and a pinch of salt to it.
  Take it twice daily.

- Mash 1 ripe banana and add ¼ teaspoon of nutmeg powder.
  Take it twice daily.

- Make a paste of 15 fresh curry leaves mixed with 1 teaspoon of honey.
  Consume it.

- Eat 4 ½ lbs. of apples a day for 3 – 5 consecutive days. Water may be drunk. The apples may be eaten raw, as applesauce, baked or cooked but without additional sweeteners.

- Eat the prickly pear fruit, rinse it very well to remove the prickles.

- Eat boiled or grated carrot as part of the meal.

- Have raw garlic with meals.

- Avoid dairy products during that period.

HYDROTHERAPY TREATMENTS

COCONUT OIL PACKS

An oil soaked cloth usually hot and placed over the abdomen. Will assist in elimination, good for headaches and constipation.

Items needed:

Coconut oil
Cotton flannel cloth
Plastic sheet
Bath towel
Two safety pins
Hot water bottle

Method:

1. Fold the flannel in two layers wide and long enough to cover and wrap around the area if need to.
2. Soak the flannel with warm coconut oil but not dripping. Put it on the abdomen, cover with the plastic.
3. Wrap a towel around the area and fasten it with safety pins. A hot water bottle can be placed on it.
4. Leave it on for at least 8 hours. Wash off with 2 teaspoons of baking soda to 1 quart of water.
   Use it every day with one day off each week and week 4 off, it can be repeated until improvement.

COLD SITZ BATH

This treatment is good for constipation, bed wetting, bladder inflammation, pelvic circulation and inflammation.

Items needed:

1 basin or tub which is large enough for the person to sit in.
2 small basins, 1 for the feet and 1 for the compress.
2 washcloths for the head compress.
Ice

Procedure:

1. Sit in a tub or basin of ice cold water up to the waist for 1-5 minutes.
2. Place the feet in a small basin of hot water or wrap them in hot towels.
3. Apply a cold compress to the forehead, constantly changing it.
4. At the end of the treatment take a 1 minute cold shower or a short cold rub with a cold towel in the area which was covered by the hot water. Dry thoroughly.

Other Book Titles by the Same Author

Can be viewed at this link:
http://www.amazon.com/author/monicasidoine

Home Remedies For Cancer

Home Remedies For Losing Weight

Home Remedies For Blood Pressure and Diabetes

Home Remedies For Headaches and Insomnia

Home Remedies For Sinusitis and Tonsillitis

Home Remedies For Stress, Depression and Anxiety

Home Remedies For Asthma and Bronchitis

Home Remedies For Dehydration and Vomiting

Home Remedies For Pneumonia and Tuberculosis

NOTES

NOTES

NOTES

NOTES

System

www.ingramcontent.com/pod-product-compliance
Lightning Source LLC
Chambersburg PA
CBHW072023290526
45787CB00014B/1769